The Many **Amazing** Medical Things
You Can Do to Tape Yourself Together

# DUCT TAPE
# 911

## James Hubbard, MD, MPH
### The Survival Doctor

ISBN 978-0-9915119-0-7

Publisher:

Hubbard Publishing, LLC

Editor:

Leigh Ann Hubbard

Designer:

Deana Riddle

To my grandson, Michael.

# IMPORTANT CAUTION—PLEASE READ THIS!

# Contents

# Tape Your Eyes

# Tape Your Clothes

# Tape Your Life

# WHY I LIKE DUCT TAPE

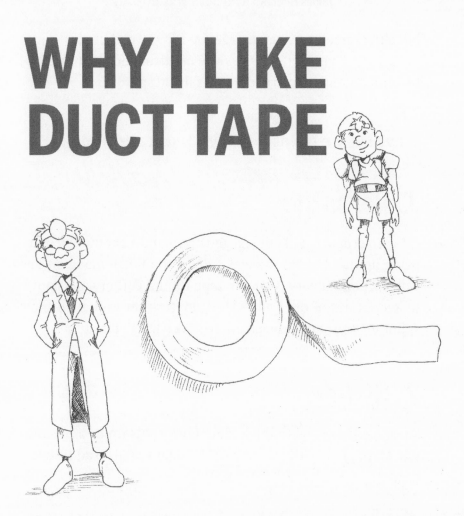

In 2011, when I launched my blog TheSurvivalDoctor.com, I set out to share over a quarter-century worth of medical know-how with nonmedical people. Believing lifesaving information shouldn't be reserved for those in the medical profession, I wanted everyone to be able to learn how to survive medical problems during disasters and other times they couldn't get expert help.

But after all those years in family practice, treating all kinds of patients with all kinds of sophisticated equipment—in big cities, small towns, emergency rooms, and clinics—one of the most versatile makeshift medical tools I'd end up recommending to my readers was duct tape.

Why? Let me count the ways. Duct tape is so:

# 1. Versatile

After you repair your cut leg, you can tear off another strip to patch up that hole in the wall. When you finish making that waterproof bandage, you can tape up the cuff of your pants to keep it out of the floodwater too. Or after taping on that splint for your arm, you can make the sling to put it in.

# 2. Strong

Since it's three layers thick, duct tape holds up to most any job. All you have to do to make it stronger is add an additional strip.

# 3. Easy to Tear

Even though it's strong, almost anyone can tear it. And because of its middle layer of mesh, it tends to tear in a straight line.

# 4. Easy to Shape

Because the tape comes in a wide roll and is so easy to tear, you can fold or shape it into about any size you need.

# 5. Sticky—More Than Most

The adhesive sticks firmly to most materials and has a stronger seal than many other tapes.

# 6. Waterproof

The outside layer is made of plastic, which keeps out moisture.

# What Is Duct Tape Made Of ?

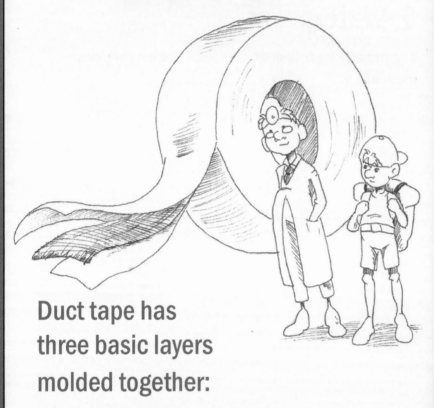

Duct tape has
three basic layers
molded together:

1. A plastic, waterproof outside

2. A cloth middle

3. An inner *rubber* adhesive **(those allergic to latex should avoid it)**

# TAPE
# YOUR
# JOINTS

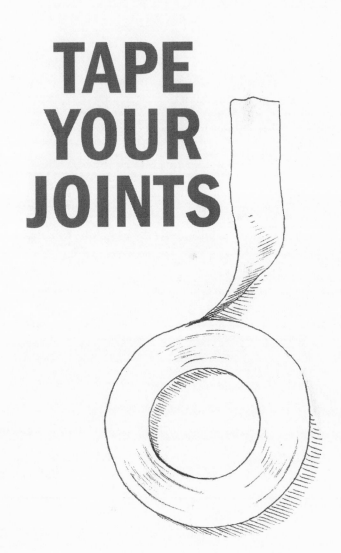

# 1

# Ankle Brace

Splints and braces are used to immobilize injured joints, hopefully preventing further injury and minimizing pain. They're firm and, if possible, moldable, conforming to the area.

For an ankle brace, an elastic bandage is an example of moldable and would do with a mild sprain. A board is on the extreme side of firm and could be the best option with an obvious break. But if you have nothing better, you can also make an entire ankle brace out of duct tape.

If you're going to be on your feet with that hurt ankle, swelling may be a problem and could cut off circulation through the duct tape brace, so don't tape the toes, and check them periodically for numbness or discoloration. Loosen the tape if you have concerns. Wearing a sock under the tape could help prevent a cut-off of circulation. If you're wearing boots, an even better method would be to apply the tape while the boot is still on.

If you suspect a break, the more you can stay off your feet the better anyway to avoid further damage. If you must walk, make some crutches or a cane out of a thick stick.

## Option 1: Figure-of-Eight Brace

I prefer this method if the victim is wearing a boot or sock the tape can wrap around.

### 1. Wrap a strip of tape above the ankle.

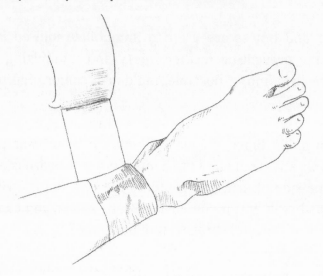

### 2. Cross down to wrap around the arch of the foot.

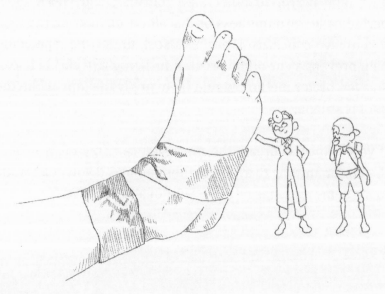

3. Extend another wrap to just before the toes.

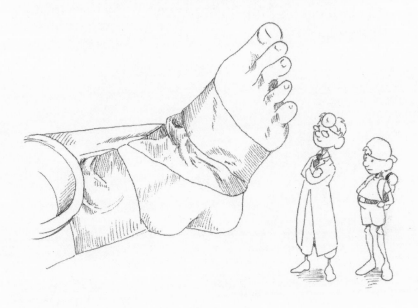

4. Now wrap back up and cross the ankle again.

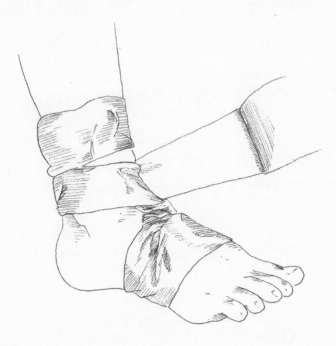

5. Continue wrapping around the ankle and foot until the brace feels firm—in other words, it's hard to move the ankle.

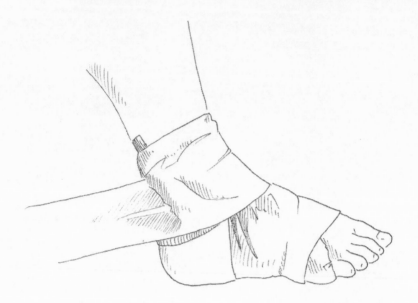

## Option 2: Ankle Splint

I like this better if you don't have a boot or sock.

1. Wrap around the ankle, and tear the tape.

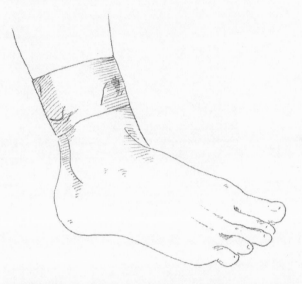

2. Tape strips from one side of the ankle and under the foot to the other side.

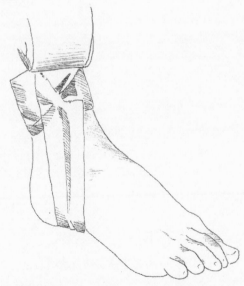

3. In the same manner, overlap several strips under the arch of the foot.

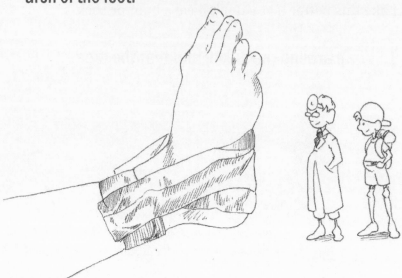

# 2

# Knee Brace

A knee brace must go from the thigh to the lower leg. As with all extremity wraps, monitor circulation by watching for discoloration and numbness below the brace. If you notice any, loosen the brace.

If you suspect a break or the knee is particularly unstable, you may need a couple of sticks on each side or a wrap of heavy cloth around the knee underneath the tape. Make some crutches or a cane if you're going to be walking.

1. Wrap a strip of tape a few inches above the knee and one a few inches below it.

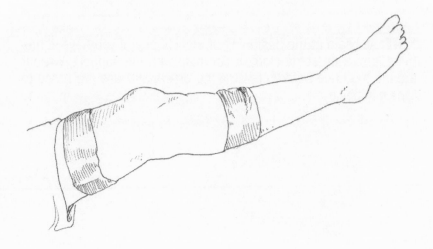

2. Connect those strips: The knee should be straight or slightly bent. On one side of the leg, apply tape from one strip to the other. Do the same on the other side of the leg. Or, if you prefer, use two crossed strips on each side.

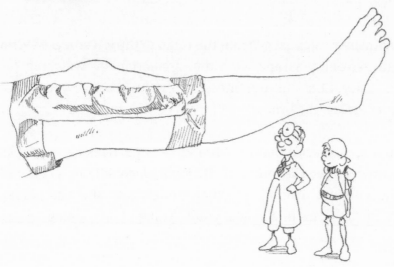

3. Apply more strips of tape, down each side.

NOTE: As I said at the beginning of this chapter, if you have something firm, even some cloth, it can help with the support. Wrap it around the knee before creating the brace, and use the brace to tape it in place.

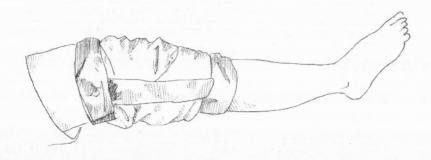

# 3

# Wrist Splint

When using a makeshift splint, as with a brace, you may have to choose between making it firm and moldable.

Duct tape is by nature moldable. And piling on multiple strips makes it firm, though still not as stiff as taping over a short two-by-four board or, say, a tree branch cut to size. What you choose to make your splint should depend on the injury and your needs. For a light sprain, perhaps moldable would be better. For an obvious broken bone, you want the splint to be very firm.

For a wrist injury, the splint should extend from the forearm to the hand.

1. Tear a strip of tape that runs from where the palm joins the fingers to the underside of the forearm about an inch or two from the elbow crease.

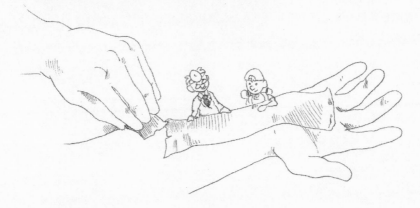

2. Tape another piece the same length to the side of the first piece to give the splint more breadth.

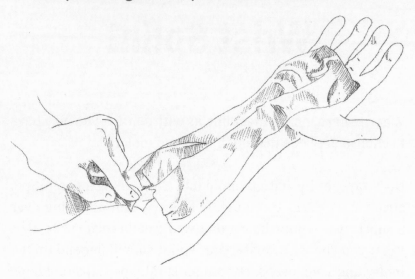

3. Remove the strips from the arm. Tape layers on top of both strips until you're comfortable the splint is firm enough. (See this chapter's introduction for more on that.) Tape a layer on the other side so the splint won't be sticky.

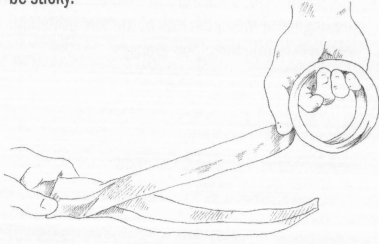

4. Place the newly formed splint in the correct position, and tape it down securely (though not tight enough to cut off circulation).

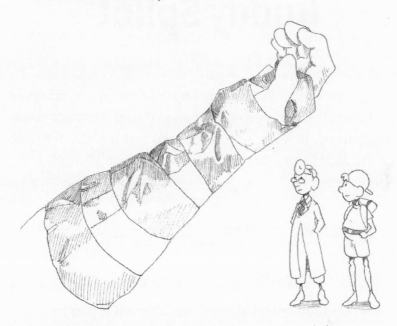

# 4

# Buddy Splint

A buddy splint is useful for any finger or toe injury, whether it be a sprain or a broken bone. It gives the injured digit some protection while keeping it functional and mobile. You just tape the digit to an adjacent, noninjured "buddy" digit.

## Caveats:

- A buddy splint should not be used if you're trying to keep the digit completely still, such as on a unstable broken bone. For that, you use something firmer, like a stick or piece of metal, taped to the injured finger.

- You'll have to make adjustments for a buddy splint to work on a thumb injury. (See the next chapter.)

1. Tear off a strip of tape about 3 inches long.

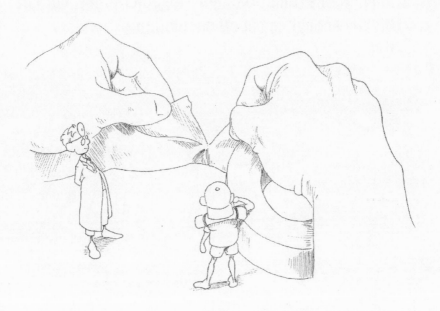

2. Tear that piece lengthwise into two thinner strips, each about an inch wide.

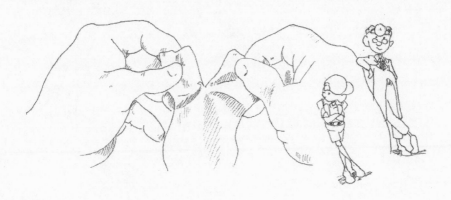

3. Place the adjacent, uninjured digit next to the injured one, and tape them together firmly, but not tightly enough to cut off circulation.

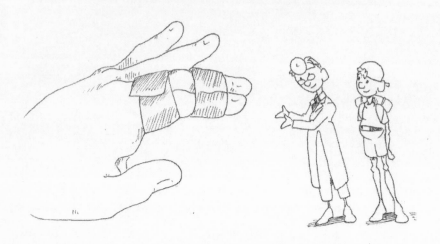

For the toes, the process is the same.

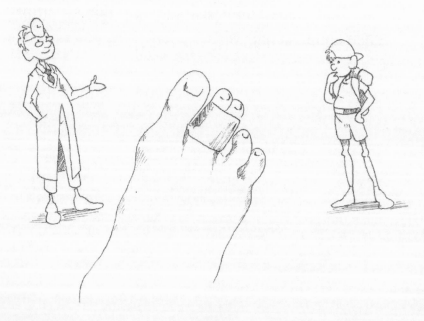

# 5

# Thumb Splint

The thumb is a special digit. Unlike the other fingers, it kind of sits in its own separate spot, and it has two additional movements the others don't have: opposition (forming a pinch with your little finger) and apposition (moving in the opposite direction).

A splint that works great on the rest of your fingers won't work as well on the thumb. So here are some tricks you can try.

As with the buddy splint, beware of cutting off circulation with these techniques, and if the bone or joint is unstable consider taping a stick or other firm object on instead.

## Option 1: Thumb Version of a Buddy Splint

This option can secure an unstable thumb in place of taping on a stick or metal splint. However, it severely limits the thumb's motion so may not be your first choice for a stable injury.

1. Wrap tape once around the wrist. Don't tear the strip all the way off. Instead, tear it halfway across. (This way, in step 2, you'll be be taping with a strip that's half as wide.)

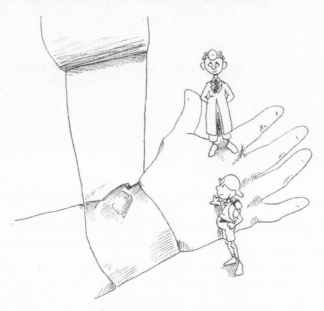

2. Continue wrapping the tape, this time diagonally across the back of the hand, up to between the index and middle fingers.

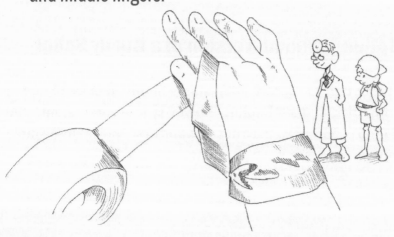

3. Secure the thumb to the finger: wrap the strip around the top half of the thumb and the bottom of the index finger.

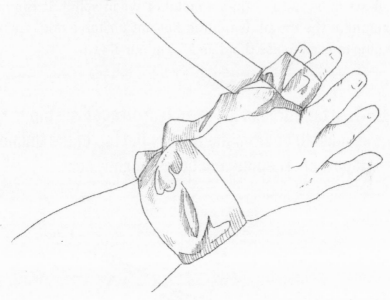

4. Secure the bottom half of the thumb: wrap the tape around it, then all the way around the hand.

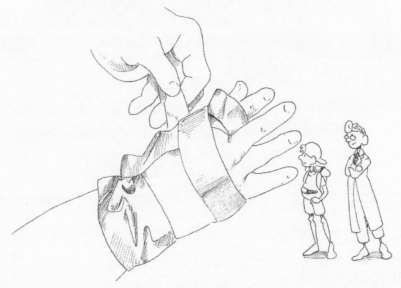

## Option 2: Flexible Finger Splint

This option provides some protection against movement but allows more motion than a metal or wood splint. It can be helpful if the thumb is injured but not unstable and you're going to need to use that hand for minimal grip.

1. Wrap tape around the wrist. Tear off another strip long enough to go from the wrist to the top of the thumb. Tape it on, keeping your thumb slightly bent.

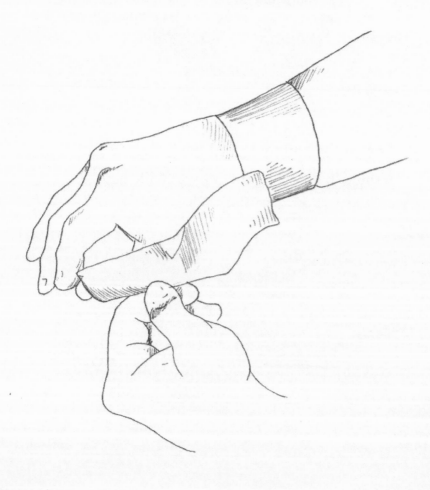

2. Tape several more strips across the back of the thumb, down to the wrist, to give the tape a splint-like firmness.

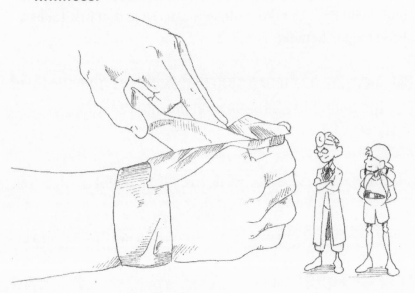

3. Wrap tape around the bottom of the splint-like strips to secure them to the wrist.

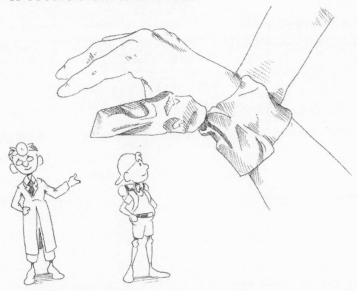

## Option 3: **Removable Splint**

This is similar to option 2, but it might not pinch as much, and if you have to take it off, you can reuse it. It just takes a little longer to make.

1. Measure and tear a strip that stretches from the tip of the thumb to about an inch beyond the wrist.

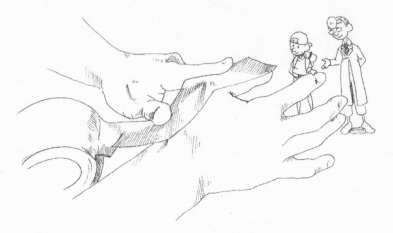

2. Tape another strip to it that's the same length, sticky sides together.

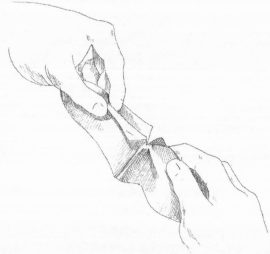

3. Tape about 10 or 15 more strips to the ones you already have, and use this as your splint.

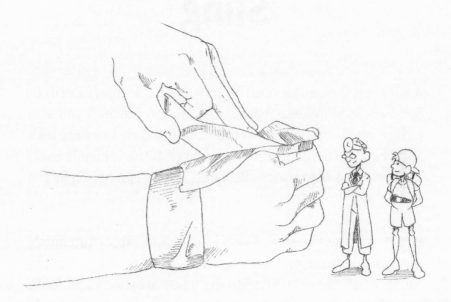

Tape the splint to the thumb.

# 6

# Sling

A sling has a number of uses. It can hold an injured arm or hand in place to keep it from moving too much. It can also reduce swelling and pain in the hand if you tie the sling high and keep the hand around heart level. If the injury is to an upper arm, shoulder, or collarbone, a sling can help take the weight off it.

Be careful that the sling doesn't bend your elbow too much, especially if the injury is around that area. Any extra swelling could cut off the circulation to the lower arm and hand. With most slings you want your elbow at about a 90-degree angle (a little more bent if you're trying to decrease swelling), give or take a few degrees of adjustment for comfort. And make sure the sling doesn't irritate your neck. Keeping your collar or a piece of cloth between the sling and your skin can help.

## Option 1: Shirt Sling

1. Take your shirttail and wrap it up around the injured arm.

*Next page . . .*

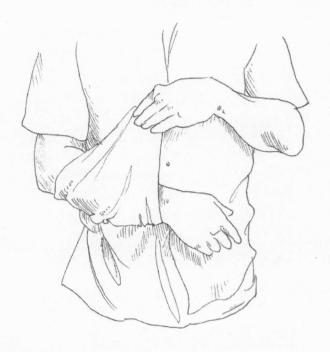

2. Tape the shirttail to the shirt above the arm.

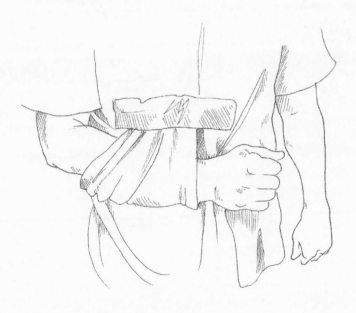

## 3. Reinforce with more tape.

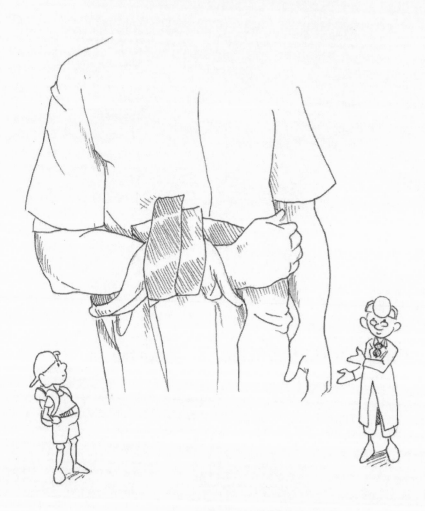

## Option 2: Tape Sling

1. Measure the length of tape you'll need to make the sling—long enough to make a circle around your neck and bent forearm.

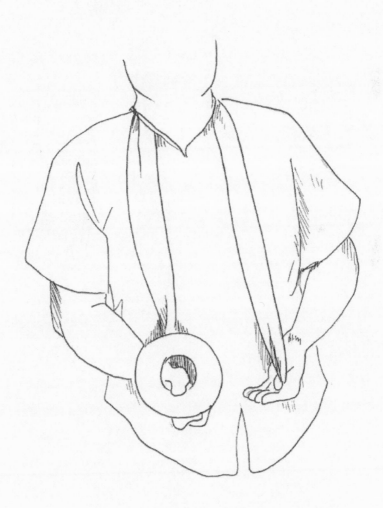

2. Tape another strip to the one you just made, sticky side to sticky side, and tape the ends together to make that circle.

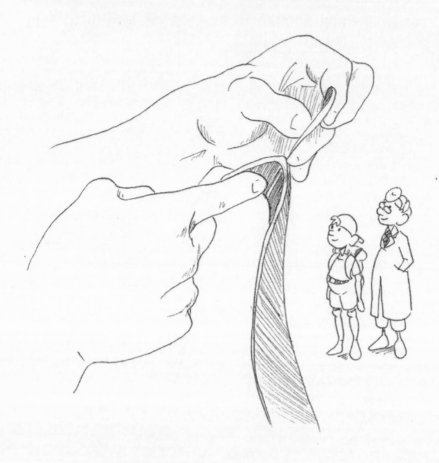

3.  Loop the sling around your neck, and insert your arm.

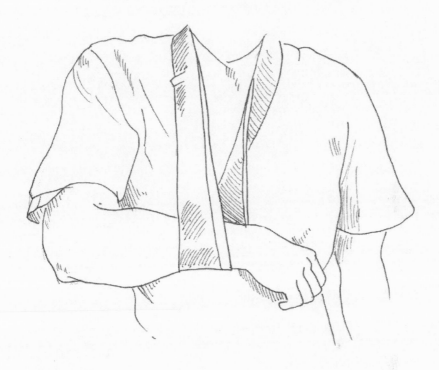

# TAPE YOUR SKIN

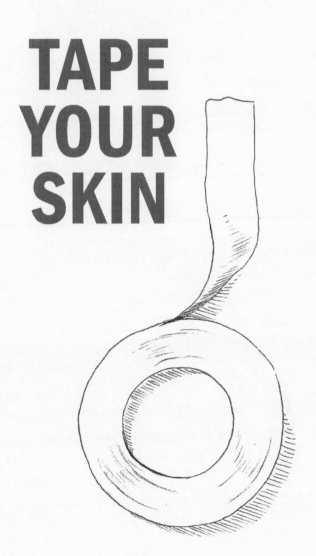

# 7
# Wound-Repair Strips

In clinics and emergency rooms, doctors tape wounds together all the time with sterile tape called butterfly bandages or Steri-Strips. This can work as well as stitching if the wound is a fairly small, shallow cut—say an inch or less long—and not over a joint (where it can be stressed) or on a sweaty palm or foot. If you have no better option, duct tape can work too.

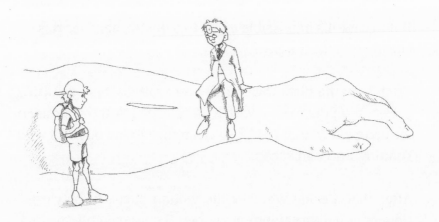

We doctors probably like to use tape on face cuts more than anywhere else. The face has such a great blood supply that the cuts usually heal pretty fast. After about five to seven days the wound has healed enough that the tape can come off. Oh, and tape doesn't cause those railroad-track scars that stitches occasionally can.

If tape works so well, why go to a doctor? Well, of course, a doctor has a little more experience than you in this closing-a-cut stuff. Plus, closure is just one part of the assessment and treatment process. A doctor has to make certain the wound hasn't damaged any blood vessels, nerves, or tendons, and decide the best way to close the wound. (Sometimes it's better not to close it at all.)

The doctor also has to make sure the wound is cleaned out well and decide how best to do that to prevent a potentially life-threatening infection. And a doctor knows better when the wound has healed enough that the tape can come off. (Tip: pull tape off slowly and horizontal or diagonal to the cut. If you rip it off vertical to the cut, the wound is more likely to come apart.)

But in case it's impossible to get to a doctor, here are tips on closing with duct tape.

First, stop the bleeding. Usually, you can do this by putting pressure on the wound with a piece of gauze and your hand for up to a few minutes. Then clean the wound out well with running water and soap.

After that, decide whether the wound needs to be closed. Generally, if it's a gaping cut, it does. If it's a puncture wound, such as a stab, we don't usually close those, partly because bacteria could be hiding deep in there and cause infection. These are very general guidelines, and they won't always keep you out of trouble. For the best and safest results, learn more wound treatment details before attempting to close one.[1]

---

[1] One place to learn more is at my website, TheSurvivalDoctor.com. More detailed instructions are available in my e-book *The Survival Doctor's Guide to Wounds.*

1. Tear off a strip of duct tape about 3 inches long. It's better for it to be too long than too short; once the strips are on your skin, you can always tear them more to size.

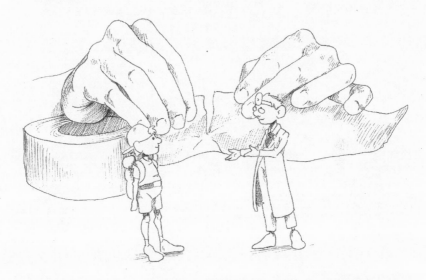

2. Split the 3-inch strip lengthwise into more narrow strips about ¼ inch wide. You'll need about two of these skinny strips per inch of cut.

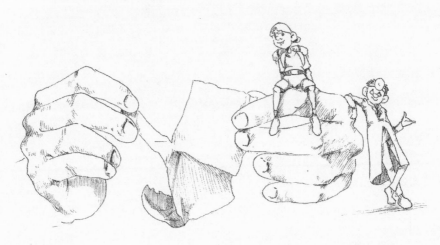

3. Stick the ends of the skinny strips to whatever's available so you can get them quickly with one hand.

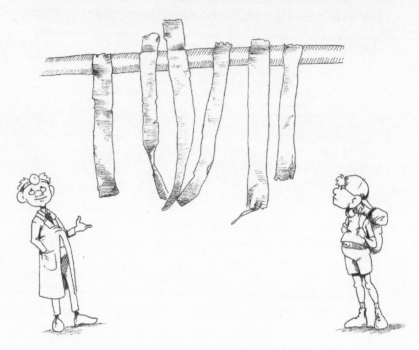

4. Dry the skin around the wound.

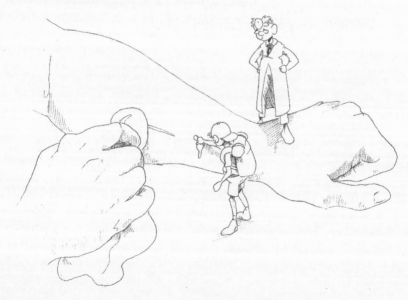

5. Starting at one end of the cut, stick half of the length of the tape to one side of the cut.

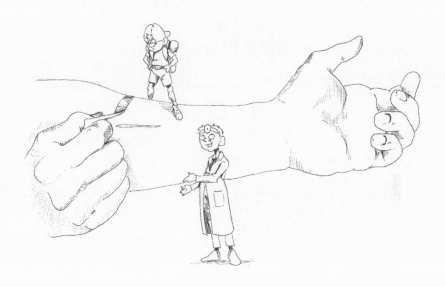

6. Bring the cut together with your hand.

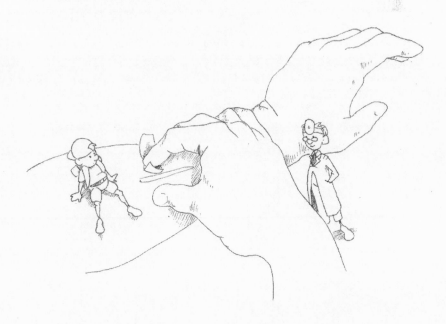

7. Tape the rest of the strip down on the other side of the cut.

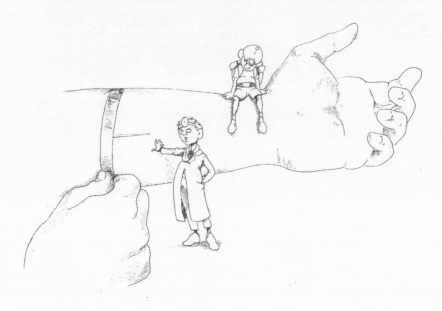

8. Position the next strip about ¼ inch from the previous one.

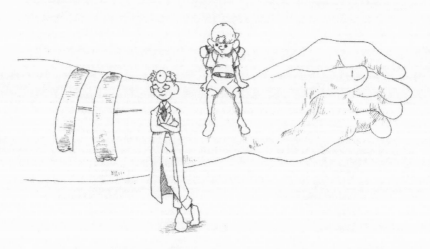

9. Repeat this process until the wound is completely closed.

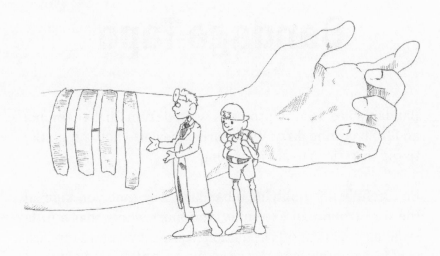

10. Apply a dressing, being careful its tape doesn't stick to the tape that's keeping the wound closed.

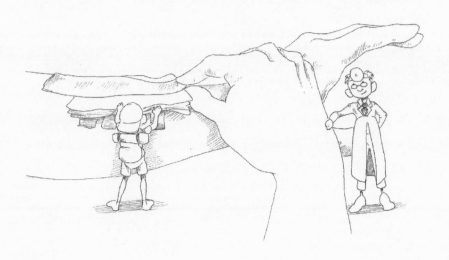

# 8

# Bandage Tape

Bandages are used to protect a wound from further trauma and from getting dirty. With burns, they also help retain the tissue secretions to aid in healing.

Be careful when applying a bandage. Any time you tape all the way around an extremity, you must worry that a little swelling might cut off circulation. For most wounds, the best way to avoid this is to not wrap the tape all the way around the arm or leg in the first place. If you do have to do a full wrap, periodically monitor the toes or fingers for numbness or discoloration. If you have concerns, loosen the tape.

1. To make your own bandage, you can use clean gauze or cloth. Unless the dressing needs to be waterproof, tape only the sides of the gauze or cloth so the wound can get a little air.

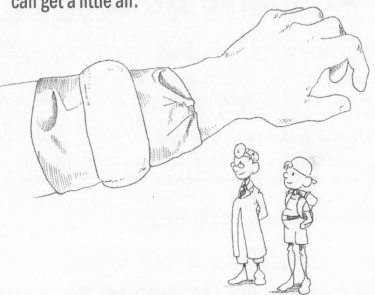

2. If you're afraid the wound will get wet, cover the entire bandage with tape.

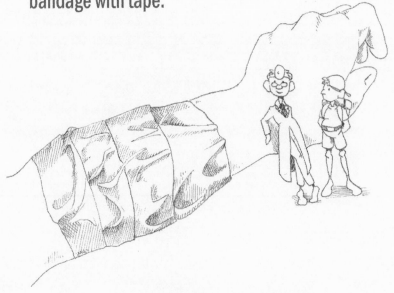

# 9

# Adhesive Bandages

Adhesive bandages are so handy for scratches and small cuts that you should always keep a few around. But, then, things tend to not be available when you need them most. If you can't find one or don't have quite the right size, they're easy to make.

First, even with a small, superficial wound, remember to clean it well. And, if you have some, apply antibacterial ointment on the wound or dressing.

1. Estimate the size you'll need, and tear the tape accordingly.

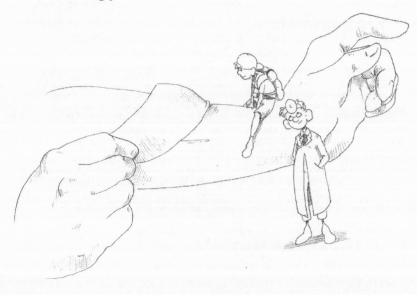

2. Cut, tear, or fold regular or nonstick gauze, or a clean cloth, to the correct size. Use enough material to cover the entire wound so you won't have tape sticking to a sore spot.

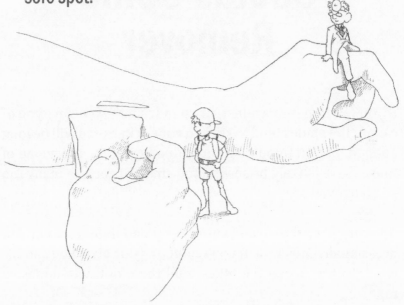

3. Apply the gauze to the middle of the tape you've torn.

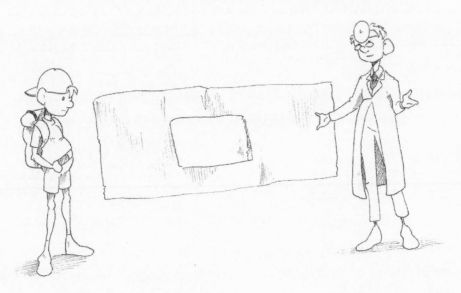

# 10

# Cactus-Spine Remover

If you fall into, rub against, or so much as touch any type of cactus, the spines tend to stick in your skin. Some will be long enough for you to pull out individually. But for every one of those there'll likely be several too small to get to—many too small to even see.

If left in place these can cause pretty bad inflammation and occasionally infection. If you're out on your own, you can try what doctors try in the office: pull them out with adhesive tape.

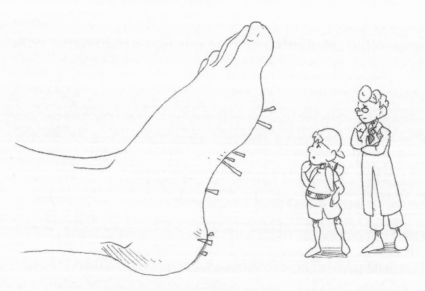

1. Pick out all the spines you can with your fingers or tweezers. Then apply a strip of duct tape over the affected skin. Press every inch of it down firmly.

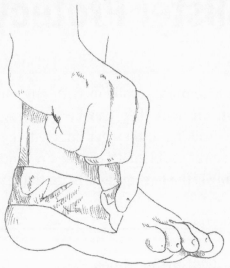

2. Pull the tape off in a steady motion. Don't jerk. After you're done, stick on another strip and remove it. You'll need to apply new tape in the same area multiple times—as long as you're seeing spines attached to the tape.

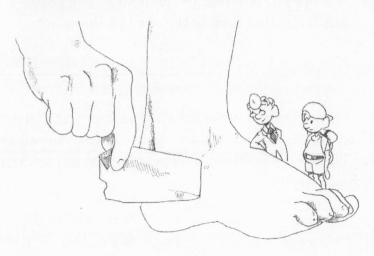

# 11

# Blister Protector

Blisters are a common problem with any outdoor activity. If they're on the foot they can be quite the impediment when you're walking. If they get infected, they can become a serious medical problem. Of course preventing them from ever occurring is the best option. To do that:

1. Wear well-fitting shoes.

2. Wear socks—two pairs if this doesn't make your shoes too tight.

3. Consider foot powder, which can help absorb moisture.

4. If there's a rough spot in your shoe, consider applying duct tape to the area to smooth it.

But even with the best socks and shoes, sometimes a blister still occurs. And if you just try to ignore it, you can end up with a big, open, sometimes infected sore that can severely limit your activities.

So if you get a blister, stop the rubbing before the wound gets worse. If you have some moleskin, cut a hole in it the size of the blister, and fit it on top. No moleskin? Duct tape will do.

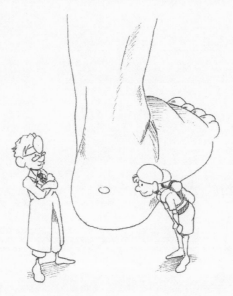

## 1. Tear a strip long enough to cover the blister and more. (Do not tape it over the blister yet.)

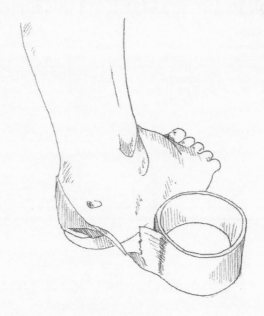

2.  Cut a hole in the duct tape about the size of the blister or slightly larger. Apply the tape to your foot with the hole over the blister.

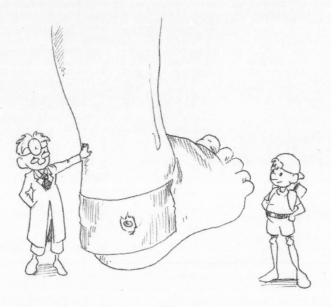

3.  Add several strips (each with a hole in the same place) to give the tape more thickness.

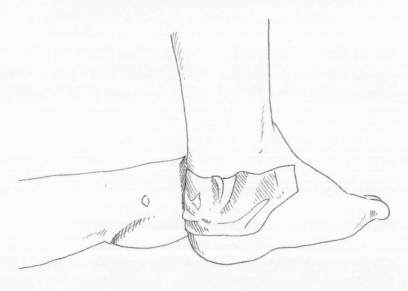

# 12

# Wart Remover

The common wart is caused by a virus. Some people are more susceptible than others. And some have one wart; others have a bunch.

Like many viruses, the ones that cause warts have no surefire cure. Left alone, they'll likely run their course and leave. But that may take years. So, many people try to get rid of warts—and try to kill the virus—sooner, either for cosmetic reasons or because the warts are in an area that causes discomfort.

A doctor can freeze or burn warts off, or you can get a wart-freezing kit from the pharmacy. But even with these methods, the warts occasionally come back because the underlying virus doesn't always die.

Many over-the-counter products irritate the warts to hopefully make the body produce antibodies to the virus and get rid of the warts for good. This is the theory on why duct tape may be effective.

One study found the duct-tape method to work great; however, repeated studies have been unable to replicate that success. But if you don't have access to any other treatment and the wart is giving you discomfort, it may be worth a try.

1. Cut a piece of duct tape the approximate size of the wart, and apply it. Keep it on six days. If the tape falls off, immediately reapply a new piece.

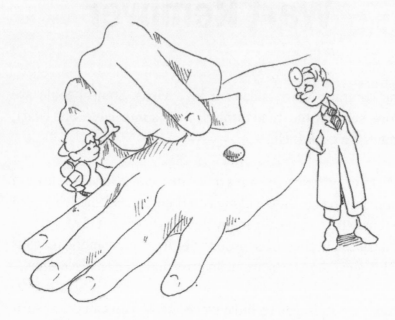

2. After six days, remove the tape, and soak the area in water for 10 minutes.

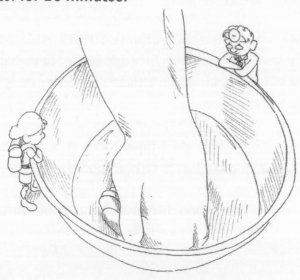

3.  Dry off the wart, and gently remove any dead skin. An emery board or nail file is good for this. (Don't file so much that you bleed; that's damaging living tissue.)

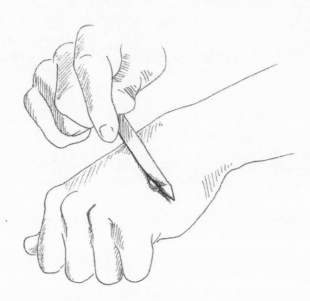

4.  Leave the area open overnight.

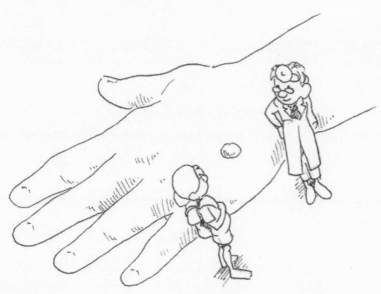

5. Repeat steps 1 through 4 until the wart is gone. If the wart hasn't disappeared within three weeks, it's unlikely it will—at least from this method.

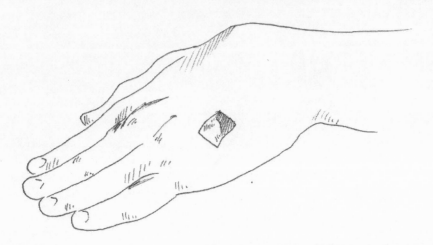

# 13

# Waterproof Bag / Pressure Cleaner

You can make a bag of virtually any size from duct tape. The bag can hold water in or keep moisture out. You might use one to:

- Hold water for drinking.

- Make an icepack.

- Store medicines, matches, or other items you don't want to get wet.

- Keep alcohol-soaked or petroleum-jelly covered cotton balls from drying out. (Alcohol balls can be used for cleaning, petroleum jelly balls for nonstick dressings, and either for tinder to start a fire.)

You can also use a duct tape bag to pressure clean a dirty wound. Fill the bag with water, and stick a large pinhole near the bottom (or just keep a tiny opening in the tape there, and hold it closed while you're filling the bag). Squeeze, and you've got water pressure.

1. Overlap strips of tape to make the bag as long and wide as you wish.

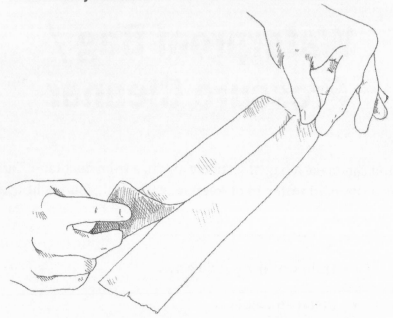

2. Tape strips on top of the ones you just put together, sticky side to sticky side.

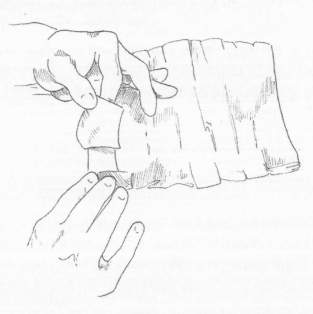

3. Roll the taped strips into a tube, overlapping the two ends. Tape the overlapping ends together.

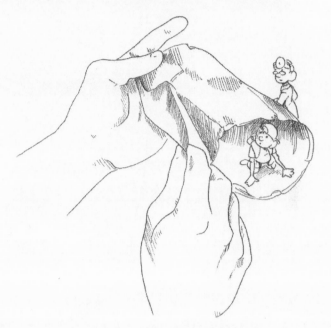

4. Pinch one of the open ends together, and fold it under.

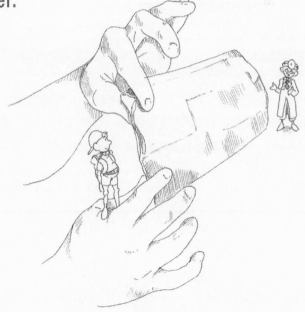

## 5. Tape securely.

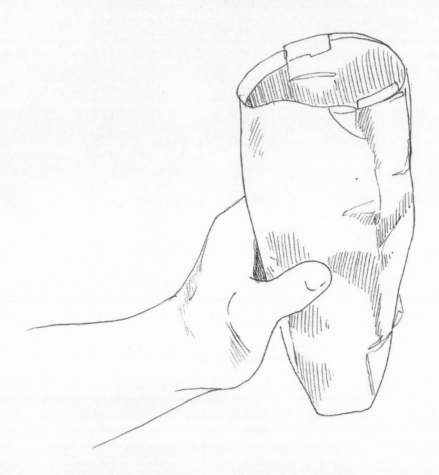

# TAPE
# YOUR
# EYES

# 14

# Eye Patch

The purpose of an eye patch is to keep the affected eye effortlessly closed. This stops the irritation that blinking causes if your eyeball has a scratch or there's something in the eye you can't get out.

Some experts think it's better to not patch the eye unless you also use antibacterial eyedrops or ointment. They surmise that with a patch, the scratch is more prone to get infected— and that it will heal better without one. Others think whether to use a patch depends on your comfort level. Most scratches heal within 24 to 48 hours either way.

Of course, if you suspect a scratch, see a doctor as soon as you can to make sure that's what it is and to get the proper treatment.

1. Layer several strips of duct tape, and fold them over to make the bulky, nonsticky patch. Cloth, cotton balls, or gauze could work for this part also.

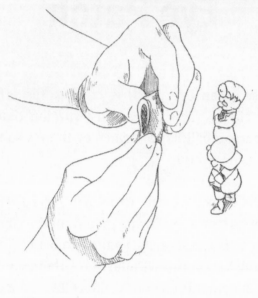

2. Place the patch over your closed eye. If it isn't thick enough to keep the eye closed, add some cloth padding under the tape.

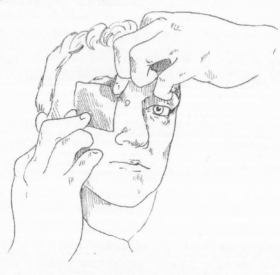

3.  Tape it in on your face (shown below) or with a strip around your head. For the latter, measure a strip of tape to go around your head, and affix another strip to it, sticky side to sticky side, so the part that goes over your hair is nonstick.

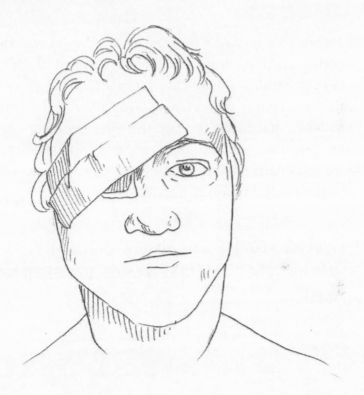

# 15

# Eye Cup

Whereas an eye patch presses on the eyelid, an eye cup prevents anything from touching the eye at all. It's used when you think you may have injured the eyeball—usually with some kind of direct trauma—or when you might have completely punctured or cut the eye. Avoiding pressure helps keep the eyeball's liquid contents from leaking or the more solid parts from herniating out. Of course, you should get expert help as soon as possible.

1. Tear off a strip of tape about 6 inches long, and fold it in half, sticky side to sticky side, to make it half the width.

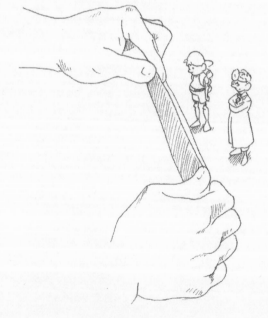

2. Roll the tape into a circle that's large enough to surround your eye.

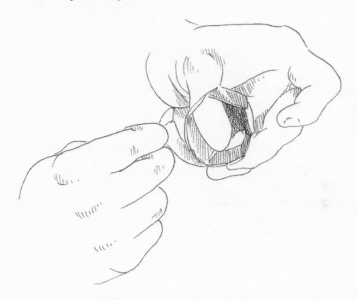

3. The tape should be touching the bony orbit, not your eyeball. It should be wide enough that you can lightly tape over it without touching the eyelashes.

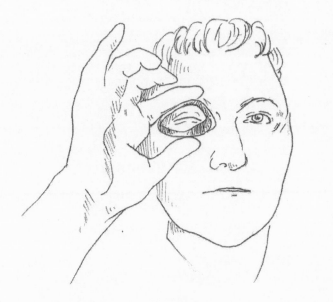

4. As with the eye patch, lightly tape it to your face or with a strip (made nonstick) around your head.

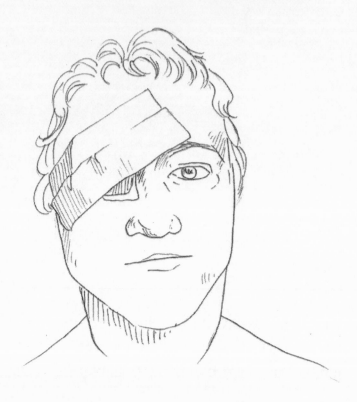

# 16

# Pinhole Glasses

I don't know about you, but if I lose my glasses and don't have a spare, I'm in trouble no matter where I am. So what if that happens when you're in a disaster or in the middle of nowhere? What if you can't tell a snake from a stick, tell a friend from a foe, or even see where you're taking your next step?

Answer: hopefully nothing if you bring out the duct tape. Put a tiny hole in it. Voilà. New glasses lens.

Focusing vision through a pinhole has been known to improve nearsighted vision for centuries. Looking through a pinhole forces your eye to take in only a small area in the middle of your field of vision. This area gets focused more sharply onto your retina (the back of your eye) than a larger field.

Eye doctors use the concept in their offices by holding a black disc in front of your eye to occlude your vision. The disc has one or several pinholes you can look through. If you can see the eye chart better through the pinholes, this gives your doctor a clue that your vision might be correctible with glasses, and they'll do more testing with various corrective lenses.

Unfortunately, the pinhole effect only works while you're looking through the hole. The claim that pinhole glasses can permanently improve your vision was disproven years ago. But in a pinch, they're a lot better than nothing.

To make pinholes, you can start with a piece of paper, metal, or anything you can poke small holes through—such as duct tape.

Of course when looking through a pinhole, your field of vision is severely restricted, but you can get around that (somewhat) by making multiple holes.

*Caution:* *Beware of excessive use in sunlight—even when cloudy—without sunglasses. Usually your pupils constrict to protect your eyes from the sun. Pinhole glasses trick the eyes by shading them. This causes your pupils to dilate and can let too much sunlight in, which can permanently damage your eyes.*

## Option 1: **Lenses Only**

1. Start with a frame that doesn't have lenses. It could be from sunglasses or your broken glasses.

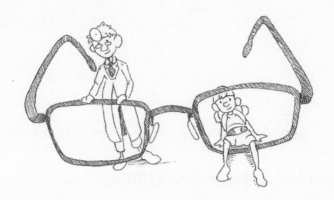

2. Create the "lenses" out of duct tape. For each one, tear off a strip of tape a little bigger than the lens should be. Punch a couple of holes of slightly different sizes into the tape. Look through each hole to see which works best. Then stick a bunch of the best size in the tape. (In the illustration, a paper clip is being used to punch the holes.)

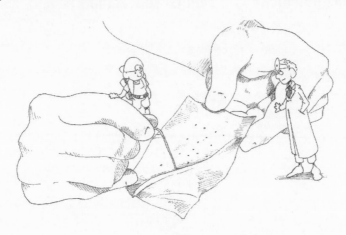

3. Stick the duct tape lenses to the frame.

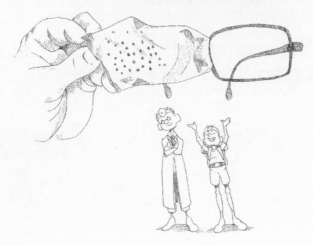

## Option 2: **Lenses and Frames**

If you don't have a frame, you can make one out of cardboard, stiff paper, frozen-treat sticks, whatever. Or you can make an entire pair of glasses—frames and lenses—out of duct tape. To do this:

1. Tear off a tape strip long enough to reach temple to temple around the back of your head. (Measure with the nonsticky side against your scalp.)

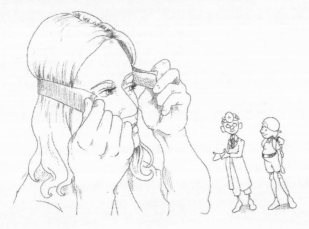

2. Fold the strip in half lengthwise, sticky side to sticky side, so it won't stick to your hair.

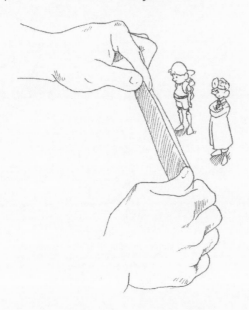

3. Set that strip aside. For the lenses and front of the frame, tear off another strip long enough to cover your eyes, temple to temple. Remove the stickiness from all but the ends of this strip by attaching a slightly shorter strip to it, sticky sides together. Leave a little stickiness exposed on each end of the original strip. Punch holes where your eyes will be.

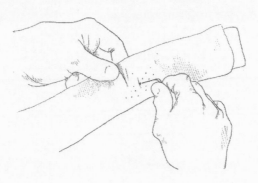

4. Cut a triangular section out for your nose. Tape this strip to the folded piece that goes around the back of your head.

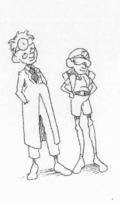

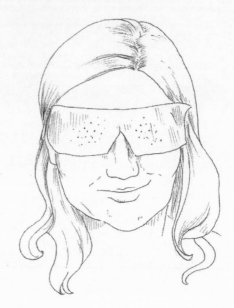

# 17

# Sunglasses

The direct glare of the sun or its reflection off the water, snow, or sand can put quite the strain on your eyes. To prevent permanent damage you can't just wear any ol' sunglasses. Now, they don't have to be expensive—that's a style issue. But they must be able to prevent 99 percent or more of both UVA and UVB rays from the sun. Don't worry, they'll come with an attached tag or sticker stating as much.

The less UV protection your sunglasses have, the more your eyes will be exposed to those potentially damaging rays that increase your risk for cataracts and all sorts of other eye problems—even burns to the cornea. Sunglasses with less than adequate protection may shade you from the visible light but not the invisible UV rays. As with pinhole glasses, the shade they add also will cause your pupils to dilate, letting even more UV rays in than you'd get without the glasses on.

Bottom line: *do not use sunglasses without proper protection unless you have to* so you can see to walk out of a life-and-death situation, such as if you're stranded in the middle of nowhere with no water, protective clothing, etc. In other words, if you're going to live, you need to leave as soon as possible—and it's the brightest part of the day. Even then, use them as little as possible.

And so it goes with sunglasses made from duct tape. They're only to use temporarily to get you out of life-and-death situations. Try a hat, shade your eyes with your hands if not full, and wear duct tape sunglasses sparingly.

As with the pinhole glasses, to make duct tape sunglasses, use any frame you have, or make one with duct tape, sticks, thick paper, cardboard, etc.

## Option 1: Lenses on Empty Frames

This is the easiest option, useful if you have frames with no lenses or if you've made frames.

1. Cover the lens areas with tape.

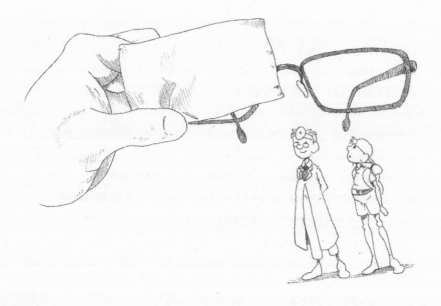

2. Cut a slit in the middle of each of your new duct tape lenses.

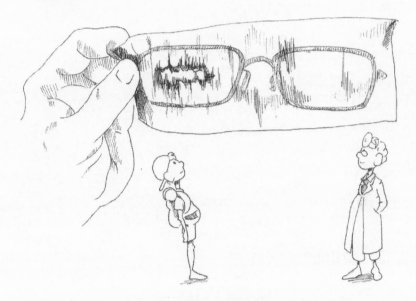

## Option 2: Glasses to Sunglasses

You can use regular glasses with lenses for this one.

1. Overlap a piece of tape over the top half of your frame.

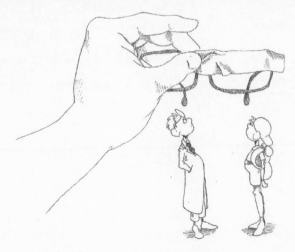

2. Overlap another piece over the bottom half of your
   frame. Keep about a ½-inch space in the middle.

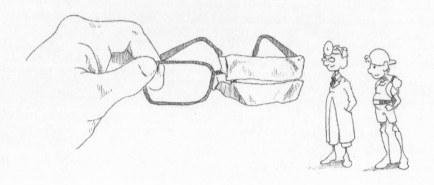

What a fashion statement.

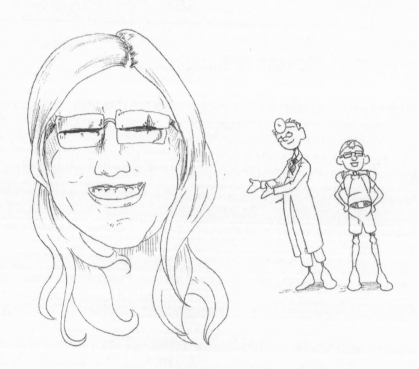

# TAPE
# YOUR
# CLOTHES

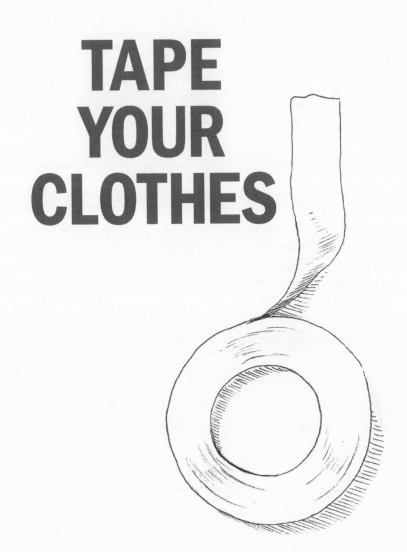

# 18

# Waterproof Clothing

Being wet makes being cold worse. Wet skin or clothing conducts heat away from the body very fast, possibly leading to frostbite or hypothermia. And keeping your feet in cold, wet socks and shoes for a long time can cause tissue damage.

Trench foot is an example of the latter. It's been a problem in wars, like World War II and the Vietnam War, when soldiers have had to stand hours upon hours in cold water. The result can be permanent tissue damage. Wearing wet socks can cause trench foot also. That might happen if you're dealing with the aftermath of a flood, for example.

And flood water poses more dangers than wetness. No matter how clear it looks, it's contaminated with whatever chemicals and sewage it's come in contact with. Viruses and bacteria can enter through skin scratches and cause bad infections. And chemicals can cause nasty rashes.

Since duct tape is waterproof, you can use it to keep moisture out of any item of clothing—shoes, boots, caps, gloves. Just tape over the item. Be sure to overlap the strips and leave no gaps for leaks.

In a pinch, you could even make your own gloves, hat, or shoes out of the tape, by either just taping it to your skin or, preferably, taping the two sticky sides together so they don't touch your skin. (Either way, duct tape isn't breathable, so it's not good for your skin; this is a temporary, emergency-only solution.)

To waterproof a shoe, wrap the entire shoe, overlapping the tape to avoid leaks. If you're going to be in water above the shoe tops, extend the wrapping to the sock or pants leg. Of course, don't wrap tightly enough to cut off circulation.

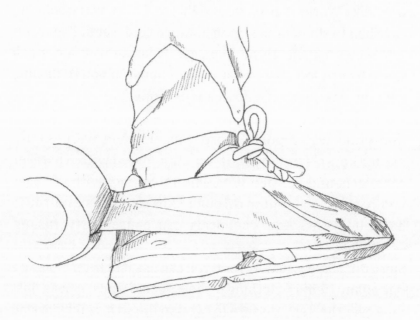

# 19

# Insect- and Snake-Resistant Pants

To keep insects, such as chiggers and ants, from climbing up your leg, close the pant opening with duct tape. This is also good partial protection from snake bites (use a bunch of layers) and a great barrier against poison ivy.

Overlap the tape strips so there are no holes, but don't tape tightly enough to cut off circulation.

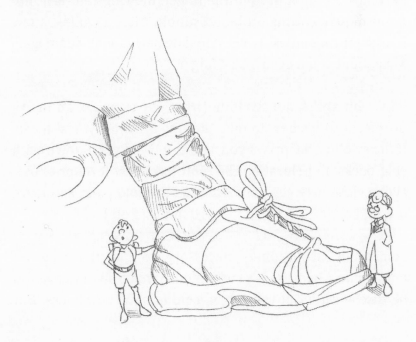

# 20
# Ring Remover

I've had many a patient come in with their wedding ring stuck on a swollen finger who's more worried about damaging their ring than their finger. The procedure described in this chapter saves both. In fact, I've had more thank-yous for sharing this procedure on my website than for almost anything else I've shared.

In the clinic, sometimes I get a hug or handshake when it works. But other times all I can offer is the reassurance that perhaps someone can repair the ring after I cut it off. That's because I've usually got to get it off one way or another. If it becomes too tight around the finger, the ring can turn into a tourniquet, cutting off blood supply. After a while—a few hours—the bloodless tissue could be permanently damaged. My patient could even lose a finger.

So, if you anticipate swelling (from, for example, an injury or infection) it's best to take the ring off while you still can. If the swelling surprises you, you can try to get it down with cold packs and elevating the injury to heart level or above. (Put a cloth between your skin and the cold pack, and leave the cold on for 10 minutes on, 10 minutes off.)

Sometimes, it becomes necessary to cut the ring off immediately because it's cutting off circulation. Hints would be discoloration of the finger, coldness, or numbness. But before you get to that stage, even if the cold packs and elevation don't work, here's one more option that might allow you to keep the ring whole. Dental floss works well for this, but if you don't have any, duct tape will do.

1.  Tear off a strip of duct tape 2 feet or more in length.

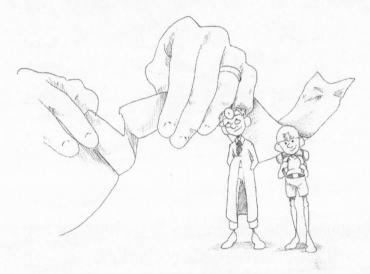

2.  From that strip, tear off a thin strip lengthwise about ½ inch wide or less.

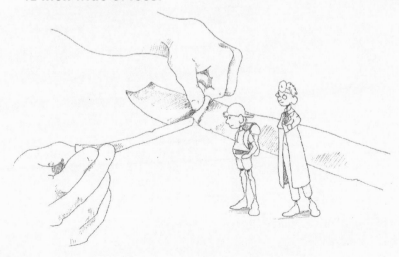

3. Fold the ½-inch-wide strip in half lengthwise, making it half as wide, and stick the sticky sides to each other. Make sure no sticky surface is left.

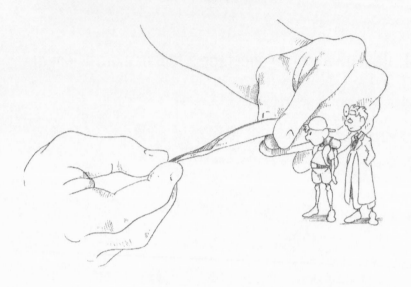

4. Lubricate the area of your finger near the ring with soap, oil, petroleum jelly, or ointment.

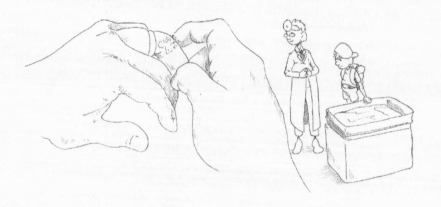

5.  Insert one end of the folded tape under the ring, and pull it so you have a couple of inches sticking out on the side of the ring that's toward your palm.

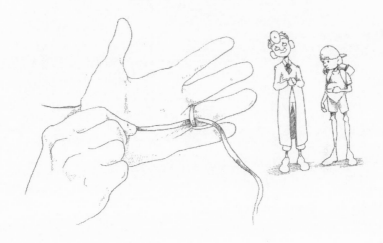

6.  Start wrapping the long end of the tape around your finger. Begin adjacent to the ring, and wrap the strip firmly up your finger past the joint. (You're trying to move the fluid causing the swelling away from your ring.)

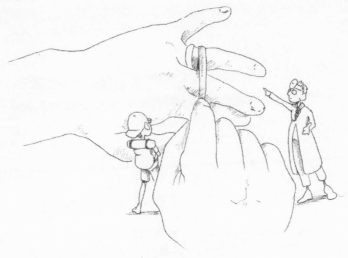

7. Continue to wrap the tape well past the finger joint.

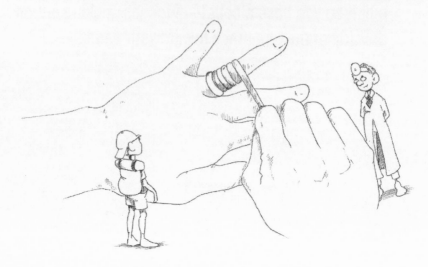

8. Hold the wrapped tape in place with an adjacent finger. Grab the other end of the tape—the one toward your palm. Pull on it, unwrapping the tape from the bottom up, as you slowly advance the ring up your finger. (It's easier if you have someone to help.)

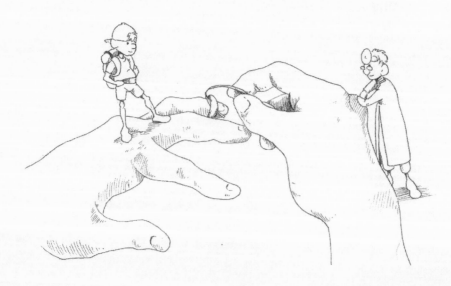

9. After you advance the ring past the swollen joint, it
   should come off easily.

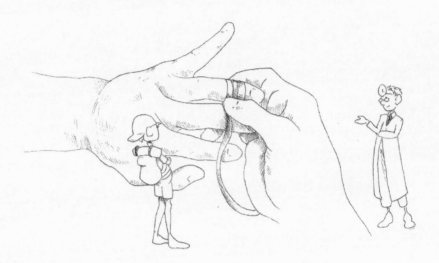

# TAPE
# YOUR
# LIFE

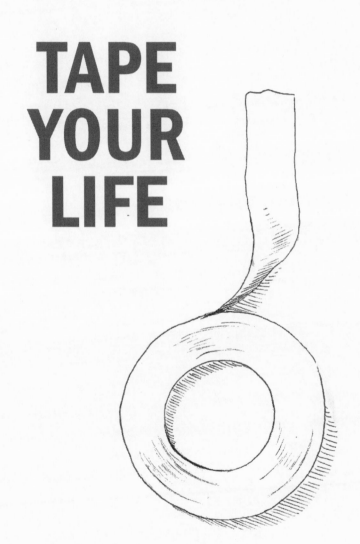

# 21

# Tourniquet

A tourniquet can save a life, but it can also be dangerous. It should be considered only with a severe wound on the arm or leg to stop heavy bleeding when other methods, such as pressure, won't work.

Once you apply a tourniquet, you should keep it on until you (quickly) get expert help. A properly applied tourniquet completely cuts off blood supply to the injured extremity and can result in permanent tissue damage if kept on for several hours. It can even cause the loss of a limb. But if expert help is on the way, current recommendations are to keep it tight rather than loosen it periodically. Remember, you're using it only if the bleeding is so bad that if you don't stop it, the person could die. If you loosen it and the bleeding starts back, it could be difficult to stop a second time.

There are commercial tourniquets, or you can make one out of a belt or strong strip of cloth. But if those aren't available, duct tape, though more cumbersome, can work.

## Option 1: Quick Fix

1. For a quick fix, wrap a strip of duct tape above the area of the wound. For the arm, that's going to be the upper arm. For the leg, it will be the thigh.

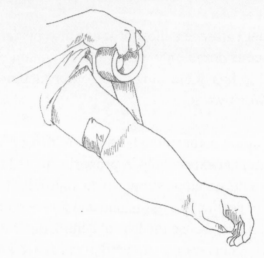

2. Continue to wrap tighter and tighter until the wound stops bleeding.

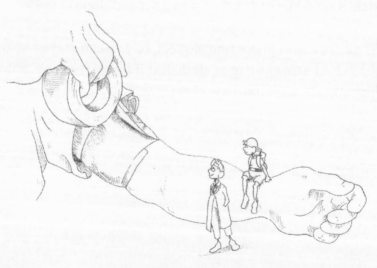

## Option 2 : Adjustable Fix

The previous type of tourniquet is quick to make but isn't easily adjustable and may pinch. This second type solves those problems but takes longer to make. If the victim is in imminent danger of bleeding to death, use the first type. This second type can be a backup if the first one doesn't completely stop the bleeding.

1. Tear off a strip of tape long enough to go around the upper arm or thigh (depending on where the wound is). Tear another strip that length, and tape the sticky sides of the two strips together. This way, the tourniquet is a little stronger, and you don't have to deal with stickiness.

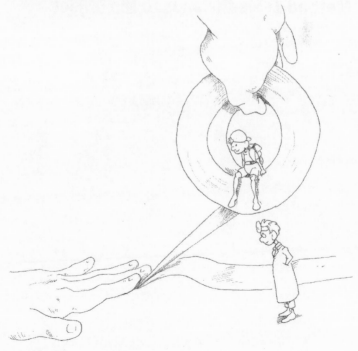

2. Find a thick stick about 6 inches long, a screwdriver, or anything of similar size that won't break easily.

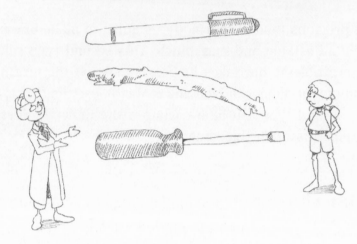

3. Attach both ends of the tape strip to the object. You can do this in one of two ways.

**Method 1: Tie the ends to the object.**

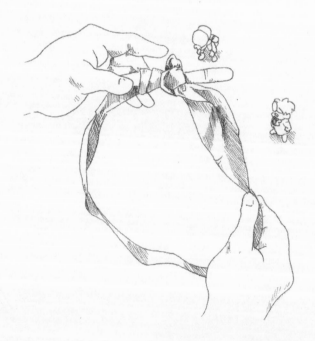

**Method 2:** Fold the ends of the strip, stick a hole in each, and insert the object through the holes. (I think this is easier than tying the bulky tape.)

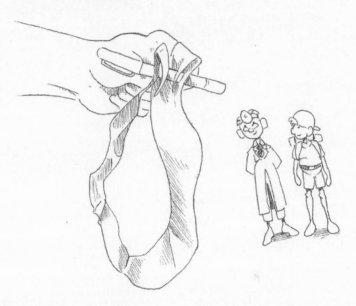

4.  Insert the wounded extremity into the loop.

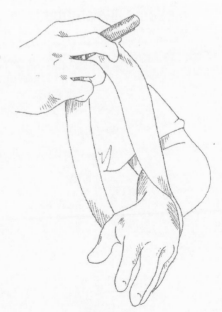

5.  Move the loop to the upper arm or thigh.

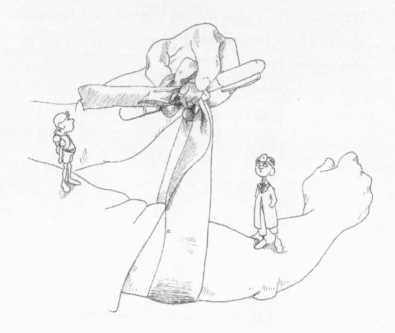

6.  Twist the stick-like object to tighten the loop until the
    bleeding has stopped.

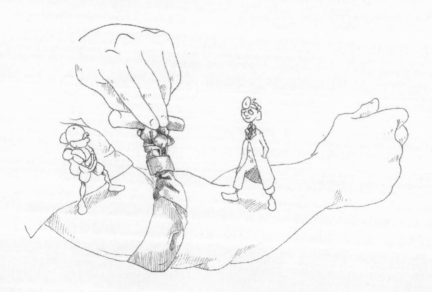

# 22

# Occlusive Dressing

Occlusive dressings are simply dressings that are airtight and waterproof. Many good commercial types are available, but when you don't have one during an emergency, you do what you can— like make one from duct tape.

An occlusive dressing can be a lifesaver if someone has a chest wound that's deep enough that it's entered the lung cavity. You'll usually know this has happened because you'll hear the hiss of air from the wound while the person is taking a breath. Or, if there's blood around the wound, you may see bubbles coming from it.

The sooner you can seal off a wound like this, called a sucking chest wound, the better because air could be entering the chest cavity through the wound and could cause a collapsed lung. Of course, sealing the wound won't stem internal bleeding or a leak in the lung itself, but it lends you some time to get proper expert emergency care.

An occlusive bandage is also beneficial with a deep burn or a wound that has been cleaned well but hasn't been closed. (Not all wounds should be closed; see the "Wound-Repair Strips" chapter.) Sealing in your body's nutritious tissue fluids can aid in healing.

One thing to keep in mind, though, is those fluids and blood can seep underneath the tape, softening and damaging the underlying skin. That's one reason you should change the wound or burn dressing daily and just one more reason you should try to get any bad wound or burn to a medical facility as soon as possible.

Below, we have an open (a.k.a. sucking) chest wound that has penetrated the chest cavity. The wound can be anywhere from a big, gaping hole like this to a slit or puncture wound by a knife or other sharp object.

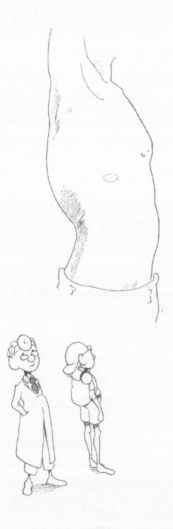

# How to Apply an Occlusive Dressing to a Sucking Chest Wound

1. If you have petroleum jelly, apply some to gauze or a piece of cloth (illustrated below) to make the dressing airtight when the person breathes in. If you don't have petroleum jelly or any other such sealant, use a piece of tape, sticky side up, as the dressing.

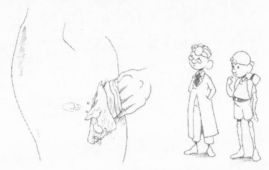

2. Tape the dressing down on three sides. Leaving one side open gives air a chance to leave the chest cavity when the person breaths out. But when they breathe in, the dressing gets sucked to the wound and seals it. In essence, you've created a one-way valve.

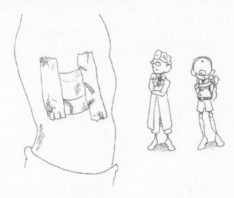

# 23

# CPR Mouth Barrier

With the various infections you can get from oral secretions these days, such as HIV, hepatitis, and intestinal infections, many people are hesitant to perform mouth-to-mouth respirations. And actually, recent studies have found that in most cases, doing mouth-to-mouth in the field (outside of a clinical setting) doesn't significantly alter the outcome in adults compared to just doing chest compressions.

So current recommendations suggest that people without advanced medical training just not do respirations in most cases. But there are times they're still recommended, like when the unconscious, nonbreathing victim is a child under the age of puberty or has a severe case of hypothermia.

You can buy commercial barriers to put between your mouth and the victim's. They have one-way valves and are better protection than a do-it-yourself barrier. But in a jam, you might consider duct tape.

1. Tear off a strip of tape long enough to fit over the victim's mouth. Cut a cross in the middle of it.

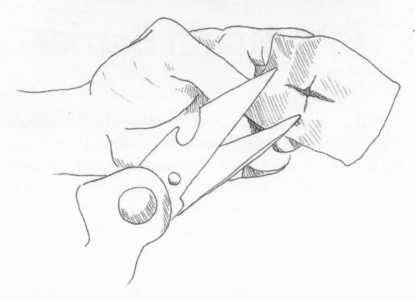

2. Tape the strip across the victim's mouth, and blow.

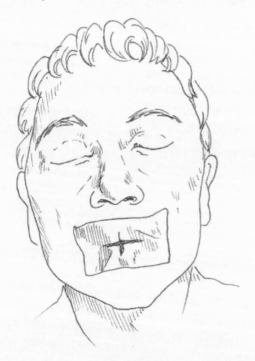

# ABOUT THE AUTHOR

James Hubbard, MD, MPH, publisher of the popular website TheSurvivalDoctor.com, is a small-town boy at heart. It was in his hometown of Pontotoc, Mississippi, where he was introduced to generations-old home remedies that got many of his patients who lived in the country, away from medical care, through hard times.

Now, he combines his make-do roots with over 30 years of knowledge as a family doctor to help other people learn to survive when they can't find professional medical help, such as during a disaster, after a terrorist attack, or when stranded in the wilderness. The tips he shares through books, workshops, videos, and his website are a combination of science, improvisational medicine, and Grandma's home remedies.

Dr. Hubbard has done just about everything you can imagine, in family care. He's worked in clinics, urgent-care facilities, and emergency rooms—in small towns and big cities. He earned his medical degree from the University of Mississippi and trained at the acclaimed Parkland Memorial Hospital in Dallas. Dr. Hubbard has a master's in public health and is a member of the American Academy of Family Physicians, American College of Occupational and Environmental Medicine, American Medical Association, and Wilderness Medical Society.

# Other Books by the Author

Dr. James Hubbard is also the author of *Living Ready Pocket Manual: First Aid* and the e-books *The Survival Doctor's Guide to Burns* and *The Survival Doctor's Guide to Wounds.* Get the latest news and information about Dr. Hubbard at TheSurvivalDoctor.com.

Printed in Great Britain
by Amazon.co.uk, Ltd.,
Marston Gate.